I0419835

Legal Notice

All rights reserved. Without limiting the rights under the copyright reserved above, no part of this publication may be reproduced, stored in or introduced into a retrieval system, or transmitted, in any form, or by any means (electronic, mechanical, photocopying, recording, or otherwise) without the prior written permission of the copyright owner and publisher of this book. This book is copyright protected. This is for your personal use only. You cannot amend, distribute, sell, use, quote or paraphrase any part or the content within this eBook without the consent of the author or copyright owner. Legal action will be pursued if this is breached.

Disclaimer Notice

Please note the information contained within this document is for educational and entertainment purposes only. Considerable energy and every attempt has been made to provide the most up to date, accurate, relative, reliable, and complete information, but the reader is strongly encouraged to seek professional advice prior to using any of this information contained in this book. The reader understands they are reading and using this information contained herein at their own risk, and in no way will the author, publisher, or any affiliates be held responsible for any damages whatsoever. No warranties of any kind are expressed or implied. Readers acknowledge that the author is not engaging in the rendering of legal, financial, medical, or any other professional advice. By reading this document, the reader agrees that under no circumstances is the author, publisher, or anyone else affiliated with the production, distribution, sale, or any other element of this book responsible for any losses, direct or indirect, which are incurred as a result of the use of information contained within this document, including, but not limited to, -errors, omissions, or inaccuracies. Because of the rate with which conditions change, the author and publisher reserve the right to alter and update the information contained herein on the new conditions whenever they see applicable.

The Ultimate Dating Advice For Men Guide!

Dating Advice For Men

Online Dating Success Secrets On How To Attract Women, Be Confident And Charismatic, And Find A Girlfriend Fast!

Ryan Cooper

Copyright © 2014 Ryan Cooper

STOP!!! Before you read any further....Would you like to know the Secrets of Transforming your life, overcome insecurities, develop leadership skills, and undeniable confidence in your personal, professional, and relationship life?

If your answer is yes, then you are not alone. Thousands of people are looking for the secret to have unstoppable confidence and self-driven power in all areas of their lives.

If you have been searching for these answers without much luck, you're in the right place!

Not only will you gain incredible insight in this book, but because I want to make sure to give you as much value as possible, right now for a limited time you can get full **100% FREE access to a VIP bonus EBook** entitled **LIMITLESS ENERGY!**

Just Go Here For Free Instant Access:

www.PotentialRise.com

Table Of Contents

Introduction

I want to thank you and congratulate you for purchasing the book, *"Dating Advice For Men: The Ultimate Dating Advice For Men Guide! - Online Dating Success Secrets On How To Attract Women, Be Confident And Charismatic, And Find A Girlfriend Fast!"*.

This book contains proven steps and strategies to guide you through the process of finding your soul mate in record time!

So all of your friends have found a girlfriend or wife and are moving on with life happy as clams. As much as you don't want to be, you sometimes feel a little jealous. Don't be, your time is on its way. In fact your time could be now! Maybe that is the very reason you came across this book. But before you get too excited, you have to know how to sift through all of the eligible bachelorettes to find the woman of your dreams.

Are you still afraid of online dating? Well you shouldn't be because online dating is no different than searching for anything else online. In this day and age of information, if you wanted to find a job, would you search for a job by knocking on every businesses front door? No, you would go online where you could sift through potential jobs before wasting your time driving all over town. If you wanted to find a house or a car, would you drive all over the state looking for a house or car? Nope, you would begin your search online so you could find what it is that you are looking for in the fastest manner. So why would dating be any different?

Here's another greater reason to try out online dating. If you're a Christian and want to find a woman with the same values and beliefs as you, it is much easier to find someone similar to you when you search online first. For instance, if you were to go out with your friends on a Friday or Saturday night, you may see 30 or 40 different women that are possible women for you to approach, but it is very difficult to know before you go out to meet them if they even have anywhere close to the same morals and belief system that you do. That's why it is so advantageous to look for your soul mate online. You won't waste her time, or yours. So don't waste anymore of your precious time, get started now! Your future with the woman of your dreams is waiting.

Thanks again for purchasing this book, I hope you enjoy it!

Chapter 1: Importance Of Shared Beliefs And Value Systems In A Relationships

"Then the LORD God made a woman from the rib he had taken out of the man, and he brought her to the man. The man said, "This is now bone of my bones and flesh of my flesh; she shall be called woman, for she was taken out of man." For this reason a man will leave his father and mother and be united to his wife, and they will become one flesh."

- Genesis 2:22-24

There comes a point in your life as a man when you suddenly realize that you have outgrown pettiness in your relationships. You begin looking for greater depth and meaning. It's not enough that you are merely attracted to another person. Instead, you want to feel a more profound connection with someone whom you share a spiritual connection with -- a woman who shares the same value systems and beliefs as you do. Someone you can call your partner in life.

The value of spirituality in any relationship cannot be understated. In fact, it is one of the things that make any relationship stronger and more meaningful. Putting God at the heart of the relationship creates a sustainable balance that allows for greater room to grow, and helps you become more mature and develop a deeper appreciation of each other's worth.

Constancy of Faith

As a Christian, it is natural that there are concepts and principles that you hold dear and strive to live up to in your day to day life. Your faith is an integral part of who you are, and you want to keep it that way. As you go about looking for a life partner, you have certain considerations in mind to ensure that you and the woman you will end up with share a mutual belief in God. This constancy of faith is something that you want to uphold in your life together with your romantic partner.

The question, however, is: Where do you begin looking for the woman of your dreams? Traditionally, you would have to go out, expand your social circle, put yourself out there, take chances, and spend considerable time trying to look for a potential mate. The whole process can be tedious and expensive, not to mention that it can only yield random results at best.

But thanks to the Internet, the world has gotten much smaller so the probability of finding your ideal partner has just become more manageable. As you will read in the next chapter, there is a science behind online dating that puts your preferences into consideration, so much so that you wouldn't have to rely too much on luck to ascertain who you will try to build a connection with.

Prelude to Something Special

Do not mind others who say that online dating is only for the desperate and hopeless. They couldn't be more wrong. Sadly, this misperception is perpetuated by those who have little idea of how online dating works and the dynamics of interaction in the 21st century.

Know, however, that online dating does not promise a fairy tale ending for those who engage in it. The truth is online dating serves only as a prelude to what will

hopefully turn out to be a fruitful and enduring relationship. It is not the be-all and end-all of your romantic life. Treat it as a crucial step to assess your priorities, find out what you really want, and forge a solid connection with someone who truly gets you.

The next few chapters will provide you pointers and guides to help you navigate the online dating terrain. These things should help you in finding your life partner and in making the most out of the experience.

Chapter 2: Science Of Modern Matchmaking

"He who finds a wife finds what is good and receives favor from the LORD."

- Proverbs 18:22

The emergence of the worldwide web in the past few decades has definitely ushered in a lot of dramatic changes in the way people do things. From education to transportation to banking and business, the world has been rendered digital and mobile by the pervasiveness of the cyber culture in modern society. At the heart of this sweeping digital revolution is the essential human need to connect and be in touch with other people. It's not surprising; therefore, that one of the first things to emerge from the dot-com revolution is online dating.

How does online dating work? The whole thing operates under the premise that successful romantic partnerships are those that are solidly anchored on shared beliefs and preferences between the two people involved. This is exactly the reason why signing up for an online dating account normally negates answering a long series of questions that range from your physical attributes to your ideological preferences. Once submitted, all these pieces of information are converted into quantitative data. These are then processed by the system's built-in algorithm, and thereafter your profile is clustered with the rest of the users whose preferences match yours.

Easy and Convenient

There are a couple of reasons why online dating has been on the rise in the past decade or so. Chief among these is the way it virtually eliminates the need to go out and spend time looking for a potential mate. The practicality, ease, and convenience that it brings appeal to a new generation of men who, because of the Internet, have developed little patience for complicated mind-reading sessions with people they'd rather have nothing to do with or share little values with.

Thanks to online dating sites, though, it is now much easier to narrow your choices based on criteria that you consider essential. The way a person looks is no longer as primordial a concern as it used to be, given other factors that you have to put into consideration. And since it's all online, you can manage your profile while in the comfort of your home or while doing other tasks. This convenience allows you to handle your time more efficiently and gives you greater freedom in managing your schedule.

Most importantly, online dating is discreet. If you are the type who values your privacy, online dating sites normally have adequate controls in place to ensure that you remain anonymous until you yourself decide to disclose details about yourself. This holds true for the other users as well. This has the potential of boosting your confidence because you are operating under an environment where harsh rejections are eliminated. Instead, the system automatically sets you up with people whom you share similar preferences with.

Getting Started with your Profile

In online dating, everything starts and ends with your profile. As such, it is necessary that your profile is able to accurately convey who you really are and what you are looking for. Similar to offline situations, you want your online persona to be taken seriously, too. Otherwise, you'll only be wasting time and resources trying to accomplish something that your heart is not really into.

Understandably, creating your profile poses a few problems. For instance, the space afforded is too limited for someone to gauge another person's values and personality. However, it is worthwhile to note that profiles only serve as starting points for a real and genuine connection. Anything that comes after that would be heavily reliant on how you handle subsequent exchanges.

In addition, the temptation to lie and be dishonest about things is particularly high when setting up your profile. How should you go about this? There is only one rule in creating your profile: Be honest. Coming up with lies or half-truths to catch the attention of others does not only reek of desperation, it is also self-defeating. Lies will find a way to catch up with you, and you don't want that to happen. You want your relationship to be anchored on truths, not lies. As a Christian, it behooves you to demand honesty in a relationship, but this honesty should begin with you.

Chapter 3: Avoiding The Pitfalls Of Online Dating

"Houses and wealth are inherited from parents, but a prudent wife is from the LORD."

- Proverbs 19:14

It would be wrong to assume that the offline rules in dating do not apply online. See, save for the interactive form of communication, the dynamics of initial interaction and dating are the same whether you are in a bar or in front of a computer. You must be keenly aware of subtleties and nuances in the way you exchange messages. Most importantly, do not forget to accord each other with mutual respect.

As far as your profile is concerned, strive for accuracy. Like what was mentioned in the previous chapter, you can be undone by your profile, so it is important that you pay careful attention to what you put in it. Fill up all the required details. This will make it easier for the system to find accurate matches for you. Remember that any item left blank means one less identifier to quantify.

Another crucial thing to consider is your display photo. This subject is contentious in that in most cases, photos lead other people to make unwarranted judgments about other users. As such, it is your call if you want to upload a photo or not. Just note that profiles without any photo are likely to be ignored than those with one.

A Face to your Profile

If, however, you decide to put a face to your profile, follow the standard guidelines for display photos. For starters, use a recent photo that approximates how you look like at present, not 10 years ago. Use one that presents you in a good light, not one that has been Photoshopped and which now hardly resembles the original version. Similarly, pick a solo shot, not one with your friends or a flashy car beside you; you do not want to deflect attention elsewhere other than yourself. And lastly, wear a decent shirt; nothing screams desperate or vain other than a profile photo of you half-naked.

All profiles also come with a space where you can write a pitch for yourself. Next to your photo (if you have one, that is), your pitch is the one thing that other users will want to look at. The key is to make you stand out from the rest. How do you do it? For one, avoid trite or boring statements. So you love animals? So do half of humanity. Avoid crowd-pleasing statements because they only make you look too predictable. Instead, identify things about yourself that make you interesting. In so doing, be brief and succinct. Do not compose a lengthy essay because that would only make you look conceited and too self-absorbed.

Grain of Salt

This being the Internet, you have to take everything with a grain of salt. But this should not be made as an excuse for you to lie. Online or offline, strive to be honest about who you really are and what you stand for. Make your principles stick out in your account, and make an effort to be consistent about them. In other words, do not contradict yourself in your profile. If, for instance, you take

pride in being a health buff but you indicated that you are a smoker, you may want to reconcile those two things by revising your pitch.

In all, do not try to complicate things for yourself. Online dating can be very direct and upfront an exercise, so it does not make any sense for you to treat it otherwise. You just need to be honest and develop a certain level of cautiousness as you go about it.

Chapter 4: Transitioning From Online To Offline Interaction

"A wife of noble character who can find? She is worth far more than rubies."

- Proverbs 31:10

Once you have set up your profile, the system will automatically present you with potential matches. These are the people whom the system figured would be compatible with you based on the things you have all put in your individual profiles. The question is: How do you go about this?

Remember that even before setting up your profile, you already have a predetermined notion of who your ideal woman is. Think about the things that constitute this representation of the ideal and use these as your criteria for narrowing down your choices. The fact that you have choices is both an advantage and a disadvantage. It can be a good thing because there are in fact people who share the same beliefs and value systems as you do. On the other hand, it can be a disadvantage because your choice would have to be narrowed down based on instinct and gut feel, and you may miss something in the process.

In choosing who to connect with, you may want to consider the distance between the two of you. Ordinarily, a 25-mile radius will work. After all, you wouldn't want to bet too much on anything beyond that. Long-distance relationships are difficult even for established unions, more so for those that are yet to start out.

Communication is Key

The key to building a connection lies in building a stable line of communication. It is through this exchange of thoughts and ideas that each of you acquires a better idea of what your individual personality is. Take this stage as an opportunity to assess each other's needs and wants, a way to gauge your compatibility. Find out about your spirituality and shared faith in God. It is in this "getting to know you" phase that you determine whether or not you would want to take the relationship further.

There are a few pointers that you should keep in mind as you keep the conversation moving. First, value brevity; refrain from composing long-winding messages that can be said in two or three sentences. Second, avoid being too self-absorbed. Make an effort to make the conversation two-way. Third, avoid initiating topics on sex. Bringing up this topic may send the wrong signal, not to mention that it may cause unnecessary awkwardness and discomfort. Fourth, do not send excessive messages. Nothing is more irritating than being flooded with emails from the same person. And finally, proofread your messages. Avoid misunderstandings by ensuring that you have your grammar and spelling right.

Meeting in Person

The important thing is to enjoy the moment and build a solid foundation for your friendship. Don't rush things. Take one step at a time in forging a valuable connection between the two of you and in building a healthy level of trust. You'll

know when it's time to take it a step further. From email to instant messaging, proceed to conversation over the phone before deciding to finally meet in person.

However, it is important to keep your expectations at bay. Maintaining a regular conversation with another person can make you develop a false sense of intimacy with her. As such, do not let your excitement about the impending meet-up get the better of you. Ditch expectations of a fairy tale ending. Be casual about it.

On your first personal encounter, make it clear that you are not a dangerous person. It is not uncommon for women to be particularly cautious, particularly in situations like this because men online are often thought to be either predatory or creepy. Suggest a public place with lots of people around. In addition, you can reserve a table in between meals so that both of you wouldn't have to stay far longer than is necessary. After all, the hope is that this will just be the first of many dates yet to come.

Lasting and worthwhile

These dates will give both of you the chance to either affirm or reject the impressions you have made on each other based on your initial exchange of messages online. If you have been honest all throughout, then there is no reason for you to get worried about anything. The key is to get to know each other better, so that not only do you learn to share things you consider essential, you also learn to put up with each other's differences.

Like any other relationships, both of you would need to invest time and emotion as you go along. This will ensure the growth and maturity of what you have going. Cherish each moment and enjoy each other's company. With a solid foundation to support your relationship, and most importantly with God at the heart of it all, there is a good chance both of you are headed to something lasting and worthwhile.

Chapter 5: Keeping Yourself Safe And Secure At All Times

"But at the beginning of creation God made them male and female. For this reason a man will leave his father and mother and be united to his wife, and the two will become one flesh. So they are no longer two, but one. Therefore what God has joined together, let man not seperate."

- Mark 10:6-9

In as much as the world of online dating presents vast opportunities to meet new people, including possibly your own soul mate, it is important not to get too caught up in the thrill and excitement it affords. Remember that the Internet is a good thing, but only if you are able to adequately control and manage it. Letting your guard down is tantamount to subjecting yourself to greater risks. As such, it is imperative that you keep yourself above the situation by employing a number of measures meant to keep your online dating activities safe and secure.

Begin by holding off giving any personal or financial information to anybody until you have clearly vouched for the other user's identity and/or authenticity. Note that dating websites do not screen nor do they conduct individual background checks on users who sign up for their service. This leaves you alone in trying to weed out accounts that you think are fraudulent from those whom you feel are legitimate. More than anything, this calls for greater cautiousness, hence the need to be extra vigilant about giving out any personal information.

Exercising Caution

Part of this cautiousness should include a few basic ways to secure your identity. For starters, avoid using your real name in your profile. Instead, come up with a username that is not easily attributable to you -- something that you haven't used yet for any of your personal or work-related emails, as well as any of your social networking profiles on sites such as Facebook or Twitter.

In addition, be very careful when using public computer terminals. Use strong passwords that are harder to crack. Choose one that includes a combination of numbers and characters in upper and lower cases. Make sure to un-check the option to remember your password on that particular computer. After your online session, log off from the site and clear all saved passwords. You can also go further by clearing your browsing history and web cache on your browser's settings.

Similarly, refrain from filling up your profile with one too many pictures. Having excessive photos on display lends a false sense of familiarity, not to mention that it makes you susceptible to being accused of vanity. Essentially, all you need is a decent, well-lit display photo. If you must add extra photos, three should be more than enough.

Dubious Online Activities

Looking after your back should include your ability to identify red flags in a particular account. In this regard, it is necessary that you develop a nose for suspicious online activities. When in doubt, remember to always err on the side of safety. This is because in the world of online dating, trust is everything

. Therefore, any hint of deception or fraud should be taken seriously to avoid setting yourself up for any form of danger. When dealing with someone whom you feel is just pulling your leg, you can remove that person from your list of contacts, block her entirely, or report her to web administrators.

A tell-tale sign of someone you should not have anything to do with is an account holder who keeps changing her username and other key details in her profile. This could also be someone who deletes her account at one point, only to reappear again under a different name. You can deduce a hundred reasons why she does this, but one thing is clear: this user may be up to something fishy.

Another reason to be wary is when a user keeps sending you spam messages or dubious external links. Worse, this user asks you to avail of certain products and services, including pornographic materials and sex-related services, such as phone sex and live chat, among others.

Domestic and Overseas Scammers

For your safety, disassociate yourself from users who seem to cash in on the surge of netizens resorting to online dating to look for partners. Scammers abound on the Internet, and online dating sites are no exception. The good thing is that they are not entirely too difficult to spot. For example, these people normally badger you for personal information, such as your physical address, your email, and sometimes even your financial information.

But perhaps one of the most obvious things in any scammer's book of tricks is the way they create fantastical stories that strongly appeal to the emotions. These stories range from dying relatives in need of money for medical purposes to fallen dictators in despotic countries whose riches are up for grabs. Most of these stories are written with little regard for proper grammar and spelling, which is indicative of the idea that these may have been perpetuated by crime syndicates overseas. Their end goal is to extract money from gullible users.

Other things that you should be cautious of are users who fake their profiles. This is perhaps one of the most common complaints about online dating, but given the freewheeling nature of the Internet, fake accounts or posers are considered a natural hazard. In the end, it is all up to your good sense and assessment of the situation if you are going to continue communicating with another user or not. But just the same, exercise caution.

Conclusion

Thank you again for purchasing this book on dating advice for men. I hope that this was able to open your eyes to a new world of finding love online.

Hopefully you now understand how incredible online dating can be if you approach it in the right way. I hope you have already begun to upload your profile and begin your search for the woman of your dreams, but if not, there is no better time than now!

I truly wish you the best of luck in your search for the woman of your dreams, and I want to be the first to toast you and your future someone, wishing you many great years together.

If you know of anyone else that could benefit from the information presented here please inform them of this book.

Finally, if you enjoyed this book and feel that it has added value to your life in any way, please take the time to share your thoughts and post a review on Amazon. It'd be greatly appreciated!

Thank you and good luck!

Preview Of:

Overcome Fear

Presentations And Speaking Guide To Overcome Fear And Shyness, Develop Self Confidence And Communication Skills, And Simply Talk To People!

Introduction

I want to thank you and congratulate you for purchasing the book, "You Won't DIE Public Speaking - 5 Easy Steps To Overcome Anxiety And Be Great Public Speaking!".

This book contains proven steps and strategies on how to overcome anxiety and nervousness while public speaking.

Your worst nightmare has come true, you just got a phone call from a friend of yours asking you to speak at her wedding as the maid of honor!!! Now what are you going to do? Just even the mere thought of doing this speech has got your hands starting to sweat and your heart beat racing.

You reluctantly agree and thank your friend for such an honor, but deep down inside you really wish you could somehow get out of this responsibility. You start asking yourself, is there an excuse I can come up with or some other way to tell my friend to ask someone else? You hurriedly get off the phone and begin to freak out!

If you have ever felt a feeling like this or similar to this, then you know exactly what it's like to have a fear of public speaking. Public speaking is one of the most feared things in our culture today. But why is it so scary, why do people have such a high amount of fear and anxiety towards speaking in public?

This book is going to help you overcome this fear and realize that there's really nothing to fear and all. By the time you finish the pages of this book I guarantee you that you will feel much better about your ability to speak in public, and not only that, you'll be eager to do so!

Thanks again for purchasing this book, I hope you enjoy it!

Chapter 1 – Public Speaking Essentials

"Fear and adrenaline are normal. When public speaking they are necessary! Without fear you would not prepare, and without adrenaline you would not have energy to move the crowd."

- Anonymous

Public speaking is a very broad concept, which has been considered a relevant human activity and skill for many centuries. Feudal lords, kings, rulers, conquerors, explorers, writers, artists, and innovators have used the power of words and gestures to win the hearts of many and overcome seemingly insurmountable obstacles. In the same way, you can utilize this instrument to show others that you can express yourself eloquently and confidently by speaking in front of a great audience.

Public Speaking is Unavoidable

Many people think that public speaking skills are not quite important because there are many instances wherein they can avoid addressing a crowd. This isn't really the case, though. As you'll soon realize—if you haven't observed it yet—public speaking is a part of daily life for most individuals. Even if your occupation or role in the academe doesn't necessarily require you to speak in front of many people on a daily basis, it's still important to be able to speak fluently and confidently.

Since it's unavoidable, learning how to carry yourself and be confident has consequently become a necessity. Confidence is an indispensable element in successful public speaking. If you want to succeed, you must have the guts to actually stand in front of an audience, no matter how small or large it may be. There will truly come a point in your life where you'll be asked to deliver a short or long message, so don't think you can just evade this possibility.

Fear is Normal

Learning and growth are impeded when fear dominates the mind and the heart. Fear is a constant companion of each and every individual and only those who have inaccurate perceptions of themselves think that they have never experienced being afraid of speaking in front of people. It's normal to be afraid because the mind uses a healthy dose of fear to warn the individual of the possible bad scenarios and the probability to fail.

People get nervous because what they're doing is important to them. More importantly, their image is quite valuable and they don't want to ruin it by messing up while speaking. Even great and famous public speakers or personalities get nervous when the spotlight's on them. Every moment on stage is unique because it's a whole new opportunity to either sweep the crowd off their feet or slip and fall through your words and excess nerves.

Once you accept the fact that fear is a normal part of public speaking, you can start growing. You can explore the next area of such an undertaking: what

constitutes your fear. Acceptance of the problem is the beginning of a great journey towards better public speaking skills. From here, you can have a better psychological setup.

What Scares You?

Fear of public speaking can stem from various elements, but in many cases, these causes are unfounded. Why? It's because they're just erroneously fabricated by a stressed mind. Your nervousness magnifies the negative, which certainly does not help clear your mind of unhelpful thoughts.

It's necessary to know what may or may not be scaring you because your anxieties or fears are not simple concerns, which you can just avoid by bottling every type of negativity up. The more you familiarize yourself with the things that prove to be adverse to your psychological condition, the better you can fight these fears off.

Thanks for Previewing My Exciting Book Entitled:

"Overcome Fear: Presentations And Speaking Guide To Overcome Fear And Shyness, Develop Self Confidence And Communication Skills, And Simply Talk To People!"

To purchase this book, simply go to the Amazon Kindle store and simply search:

"OVERCOME FEAR"

Then just scroll down until you see my book. You will know it is mine because you will see my name "Ryan Cooper" underneath the title.

Alternatively, you can visit my author page on Amazon to see this book and other work I have done. Thanks so much, and please don't forget your free bonuses

DON'T LEAVE YET! - CHECK OUT YOUR FREE BONUSES BELOW!

Free Bonus Offer: Get Free Access To The PotentialRise.com VIP Newsletter!

Once you enter your email address you will immediately get free access to this awesome newsletter!

But wait, right now if you join now for free you will also get free access to the "LIMITLESS ENERGY" free EBook!

To claim both your FREE VIP NEWSLETTER MEMBERSHIP and your FREE BONUS Ebook on LIMITLESS ENERGY!

Just Go To:

www.PotentialRise.com

www.ingramcontent.com/pod-product-compliance
Lightning Source LLC
Chambersburg PA
CBHW061949280526

45787CB00004B/1781